Zipping it Up

*How to Lose 5 Pounds
Fast
And look great in
That little black dress!*

By Irene Gabelnick

Front cover illustration and design by Kathrine Forster Kuo.

Published by Irene Gabelnick, LLC (the "Publisher")

In loving memory of my dear sister
Natalie Kernycznyj
Who always believed in me.

Table of Contents

Introduction

Discover how to feel confident in everything you wear. *Or nothing at all…*

Are you ready to zip up your little black dress? If you have an upcoming event, a black-tie dinner, a fancy wedding or maybe a hot date. Especially if you're planning a vacation and want to look hot in your favorite bikini, then this book is for you. You will learn a quick way to lose 5 pounds fast and look great in your little black dress. This book isn't for everyone. It's based on eating a high protein and very low carb, Keto style diet. If you're going to eat crap you might as well save your money. This book is for serious people who want to feel confident and look great in everything you wear.

This plan is NOT a diet. It is about burning more calories and shocking your system into losing weight fast. I don't believe in diets and you will not go hungry. They don't work. More often, than not, people who go on diets end up gaining the weight back. Or worse, end up gaining even more weight after they go off the diet. Most of the things I will show you in this book are rules I live by. Not only when I want to lose 5 pounds fast but that I have built into my daily lifestyle.

You will need to exercise if you want to lose weight using my methods. If you exercise regularly you'll want to step up your game. I'll show you ways to squeeze in more exercise even on the busiest days.

The most important thing, that is crucial to your success is your mindset. You have to actually want to do it. If you don't really care about looking good and zipping it up, then you won't do the work. Plain and simple. You might as well grab a bag of chips and head on over to the couch while you flip through the pages.

But for those of you who are serious and want to look great and feel your best - just flip the page. Let's do this!

Chapter 1
Vital to Your Success

There are two things that are vital to your success. Your attitude and your determination. I will repeat these things throughout the book. Sometimes in different words. If I repeat things, it's because they're important. The first thing I want you to do is create a visual of your goal. If it's a little black dress, hang it somewhere where you will see it every day. If you haven't bought it yet, find a picture and hang it up. A good place to hang a picture is on your refrigerator. This will deter you from making poor eating choices and remind you of your goal.

If it's a vacation you're losing weight for, then hang up that string bikini you're planning to wear on the beach. Or a picture of your tropical destination. It might sound silly but just do it. It works. I once hung up a picture of a girl running. She had a hot body and a fierce look of determination on her face. I put it right on the refrigerator where I would see it every time I opened the fridge. It will make you think twice about what you decide to eat.

If you follow my methods, you should be able to lose about 5 pounds within a week. You will have to slowly work certain foods back into your diet, so you don't gain it all back. It is my hope that you will incorporate some of these things into your lifestyle and live a happier and healthier life.

Keep in mind, this is short term. You are not giving up your favorite foods for life. You have a very set goal that is easily achievable. Trust me. You can do this. It's only a week. Just ask yourself how much you want it.

I will be sharing with you, ways to burn more calories throughout the day, how to stay full longer, healthy snacks, what types of foods you should eat and a few healthy recipes. I will also show you ways to keep the weight off and maintain a healthy weight. But these are guidelines. You're a big girl and I am not your mother. Use your judgment and do what's best for you.

Let's get started...

Chapter 2
Let's Talk Food

When I want to lose a couple pounds quickly I make a big pot of my favorite homemade vegetable soup (see recipes). It becomes my quick and easy go to food. Because it's loaded with vegetables I allow myself to eat as much of it as I want. I am guilty of adding a little sprinkle of salt into my bowl since I don't add any additional salt into the stock. I also like to add a lot of pepper. Start there if you want, but remember this is just a suggestion. You'll have plenty of choices to get you through the week.

Your diet this week is mainly going to consist of protein and vegetables. There are more things you cannot eat than things you can. I realize giving up bread, pasta, anything with flour, wheat (even whole grains), rice, sugar and fruit is not going to be easy. But again, the idea here is to shock your system without going hungry. This is NOT forever. You will have the rest of your life to enjoy these foods. You must want this to succeed.

On the bright side, this may be the only time someone tells you to eat as much cheese as you want. Go a little crazy and try new kinds of cheese. Just hold the crackers.

Preparation:
The best way to prepare for this week, so you can achieve your goals is to have lots of the foods you'll be eating, readily available. Buy what you're planning to eat. If possible, do not have food around that you will not be eating, or you'll be tempted. Obviously, this will be more difficult if you have a family you need to feed. If this is the case, you will definitely need more will power.
But trust me on this - if I can do it - so can you.

What you CAN and should eat this week:

Vegetables, vegetables, vegetables - green, leafy and colorful vegetables are the best.

High protein foods:

Lean meat
Chicken
Eggs
Turkey
Ground turkey
Turkey burgers (no bun)
Veggie burgers (no bun)
Beans
Lentils
Nuts
Tofu
Nut butter
Shrimp
Fish
Shellfish
Greek yogurt
Cheese

What you CANNOT eat this week:

Bread - or anything with breading on it (this includes whole grains and croutons)
Wheat
Rice

Sugar - any treat or sweet that is laden with sugar
(including sugary drinks)
Pasta
Potatoes
Potato chips
Donuts
Cookies
Cake
Muffins
Ice cream
Candy
Fruit
Juice
Soda (pop)
Sweet sugary coffee drinks

Important:

- Sweet sugary coffee drinks - you won't die if you
  don't get your latte this week. But it's your call and
  your body - just don't blame me when you can't zip
  up that dress next week.

- Potatoes - I realize that potatoes are vegetables
  and there is no question that they are healthy, but
  they are loaded with carbs so skip them this week.

- Fruit - fruit is healthy and should be a part of your
  regular everyday diet. They are also loaded with
  carbs and sugar so it's counterproductive if you're
  trying to lose weight fast. I do provide a list of lower
  carb fruit in the snack section. If you need to satisfy
  a sweet tooth, go ahead and have a little fruit.

- Moderation - I am a huge believer in "everything in moderation" but you have a goal to achieve. This is not a diet I recommend unless it is short term and with one purpose in mind. To lose weight fast.

- Cheating - if you cheat and must have a small piece of chocolate or a slice of bread, don't beat yourself up over it. Just don't do it again. Get back on track and stay the course. Remind yourself why you're doing this and keep going.

- I don't like vegetables laden in butter or sauce and normally I would suggest staying away from this. But this week you might need the fat. Just don't overdo it. Save it for the cheese.

Chapter 3
Breakfast, Lunch & Dinner

Breakfast is the most important meal of the day. It helps you get your metabolism going and gives you energy to conquer the day. But I'm not usually hungry first thing in the morning. I like to start the day with a cup of tea. I drink my tea black with no sugar and sometimes a little lemon.

Then I enjoy a cup of freshly brewed coffee with cream. It fills me up until it's time for breakfast. I mix regular half and half with a little fat free half and half to reduce my fat intake. But this week fat is our friend and carbs are the enemy. If you prefer a little sugar that is fine. But if you dump a heaping amount of sugar into your coffee or tea, it's counterproductive. You're limiting your carbs this week and sugar is high in carbs. So, skip it. You might find that after a few days you don't even miss it.

Whatever your morning routine, it's okay to keep doing it as long you don't load up on sugar or carbs. You can even try a cup of warm water with lemon if you don't drink tea or coffee.

<u>Breakfast Ideas:</u>
Spinach eggs with cheese
Over easy egg with cheese
Veggie cream cheese on celery (see recipe)
Greek Yogurt

<u>Lunch Ideas:</u>
Turkey burgers (no bun)
Veggie burgers (no bun)
Shrimp and avocado salad (see recipe)
Salad - any salad will do - omit the croutons
Hummus on a bed of lettuce
Homemade Vegetable Soup (see recipe)

<u>Dinner Ideas:</u>
Shrimp with Broccoli (See recipe)
Hummus on a bed of lettuce
Turkey burgers (no bun)
Veggie burgers (no bun)
Shrimp and avocado salad (see recipe)
Salad - any salad will do – hold the croutons
Quiche – with no crust
Stir fry (Vegetable, chicken, shrimp or tofu)
Homemade Vegetable Soup (see recipe)
Spaghetti squash or zucchini with sauce

This is just to give you a few quick ideas. Your options are limitless. Just follow the food guidelines and avoid anything loaded with carbohydrates.

It might seem mundane eating some of the same things day after day. But keep in mind, it's only one week. Then you can slowly bring back some of the foods you miss. But just remember that if want to keep it off, you can't go back to eating unhealthy food all the time.

Chapter 4
Quick Healthy Snacks

You should always try to keep a healthy snack in your car or with you on the go. It will prevent you from going through a drive thru and binging on unhealthy food.

Here are some healthy snack choices:

*Celery and carrot sticks - Cut them up ahead of time and put them in individual sized portion containers. This way you can grab them easily for the car before running errands or while taking a quick break from work.

*Fresh green beans - buy them washed and ready to eat so you can just grab them and go.

*Raw vegetables - any vegetable makes a great snack. Cauliflower, broccoli, baby bell peppers or bell peppers cut into strips. You get the picture. Veggies. Veggies. Veggies.

*Fruit - grab an apple, apricot, banana or handful of grapes for a quick snack. Here are some fruits that are lower in sugar and/or carbs: lemons, limes, berries, apricots, kiwi and oranges.

*Nuts - preferably unsalted or lightly salted to prevent water retention. Pack them in individual size servings to avoid eating an entire container.

*Plain Greek yogurt. Mix with fresh or frozen berries if you don't like the taste of plain yogurt. Add granola for a crunchy treat.

*Granola bars (or granola) can be a healthy snack and satisfy a sweet tooth. Just be careful of high fat and sugary granola bars. Read the ingredients and the nutrition facts. If they are high in protein they will stave off hunger. They are also packaged well so they'll keep in the car without getting stale. A granola bar will trump a burger and fries or coffee and a donut any day.

*Nut butter. There are so many to choose from: almond butter, cashew butter, sunflower butter, soy butter, walnut butter. The all-natural nut butters are best. Select ones with fewer ingredients. Try all-natural almond butter on a banana or celery stick. Delicious!

Chapter 5

Recipes

Hearty Homemade Vegetable Soup

Prep Time: 10 minutes **Cook Time:** 20 minutes

Servings: 8-10 **Serving size:** 1 cup

Ingredients:
1 tablespoon olive oil
1 small onion (peeled and cut in half)
3 cups raw cauliflower (broken into florets)
3 carrots (sliced)
3 celery stalks (sliced)
1 small zucchini (cut into large chunks)
2 cups frozen cut green beans (place in bowl on counter
    until ready to use)
1 14-ounce can whole tomatoes (cut or broken into large
pieces - do NOT discard the juice)
6 cups Vegetable stock
1/2 teaspoon dried oregano
1 teaspoon dried parsley (1 tablespoon fresh)
½ teaspoon thyme
1 bay leaf
Fresh ground pepper to taste

Directions:
Heat olive oil in large soup pot. Add carrots and celery.
Sauté for 2-3 minutes until tender crisp. I like to add about
a tablespoon of water and cover to steam the vegetables.
Stir occasionally. Add vegetable stock, tomatoes with juice
from can, oregano, parsley, thyme, onion, pepper and bay
leaf. Heat until steaming. Add zucchini. Cook another 3 to
5 minutes. Add green beans (should be slightly thawed by
now). Bring to a simmer. Simmer for about another 5
minutes or until vegetables are soft but still tender crisp.
Zucchini should be soft and opaque but not mushy.

Discard bay leaf and onion. Serve.

Variations:
*Add cooked Ditalini pasta (or pasta of choice) for a
heartier, more filling soup. We leave it on the side and add
it to our bowls so having carbs is optional.
*Add 1 can navy beans (rinsed and drained) for a high
protein variation.

Tips:
*You can cut the tomatoes right in the can using kitchen
shears.
*Adding the frozen green beans slows down the cooking
process to prevent the other vegetables from getting
overcooked.
*Let the soup cool in the pot. Then freeze half. To thaw:
pull out the soup at least one day before use and place in
refrigerator overnight. Heat in a medium saucepan on low
heat until heated through. Do NOT boil. If you decide to
pull it out and serve it on the same day, you can thaw on
defrost in the microwave before heating on the stove. Or
you can continue to heat in the microwave after thawing. It
has been my experience that the microwave reheating
method can make the vegetables a little mushy.

Quick & Easy Shrimp with Broccoli

Ingredients:
2 cloves garlic (smash or chopped)
1 - 2 heads of broccoli - approximately 3 cups (cleaned
and cut into florets)
1 pound frozen cooked shrimp (medium or large)
1 tablespoon olive oil
Pepper to taste
Crushed red pepper to taste (optional or serve on the size)
Parmesan cheese to sprinkle on top or serve on the side

Preparation:
Thaw frozen shrimp by placing in a colander and running
cold water over them (or follow thawing instructions on the
package). Pat dry with paper towels. I like to remove and
discard the tails, but you can leave them on to add more
flavor. You can thaw them ahead of time and place them in
an airtight container in the refrigerator until ready to use.

Heat oil in pan. Sauté garlic for about 1 minute. Add
broccoli and 2 tablespoons water. Sauté approximately 4-5
minutes. Add more water if needed and cover to steam
and retain liquid. Add shrimp and season with black
pepper. Heat through approximately 2-3 minutes.
Serve with crushed red pepper and parmesan cheese.

Makes approximately 3-4 servings. Makes a perfect lunch
leftover to heat and serve.

Shrimp and Avocado Salad

Ingredients:
4 cups iceberg or butter lettuce
8 ounces cooked shrimp (chilled or use frozen thawed cooked shrimp) 1 avocado (sliced)
½ cup canned black beans (rinsed and drained)
½ cup grape tomatoes or 1 tomato sliced into wedges
¼ cup shredded mozzarella cheese
Salsa (optional)
Dressing of choice (optional)

Preparation:
Divide lettuce onto two plates. Sprinkle beans and shredded mozzarella cheese over lettuce dividing evenly. Place avocado, tomatoes and shrimp around plate dividing evenly. Serve with salsa and/or dressing of choice. Makes 2 servings.

Veggie Cream Cheese

If you're looking for a great way to add more vegetables to your breakfast, try this recipe. It makes a great breakfast or snack on celery or carrots.

Ingredients:
4 ounces cream cheese (Neufchatel or ⅓ less fat)
⅓ cup chopped carrots
⅓ cup chopped celery
1 green onion sliced
Pinch of garlic powder (optional)

Mix together in a 2-cup container with lid. Will keep refrigerated up to a week.

Spicy Crunchy Chickpeas

This recipe is perfect for a healthy filling protein snack.

Ingredients:
1 can garbanzo beans (or 2 cans to make a double batch)
cayenne pepper to taste (or seasoning of your choice)
paprika black pepper
olive oil
salt

Directions:
Preheat oven to 400 degrees. Rinse and drain garbanzo beans. Wipe dry with paper towels. This recipe works best if you let them air dry for a while before baking. But if you don't want to wait just cook them a little longer. I usually remove most of the loose skin after drying them. You don't have to but they cook more quickly and might burn while baking. Drizzle with olive oil and mix in spices to taste. Line a baking sheet with aluminum foil (or parchment paper). Spread mixture evenly in a single layer and sprinkle with a little more cayenne pepper. If you want them extra spicy. Bake for 30 to 40 minutes or until brown and crispy.

* These are so delicious you probably won't have any left. But if you do, store them in an open container. If sealed, they will lose their crunchiness.

Chapter 6
Exercise - Move That Body

I'm going to take a shot in the dark here and assume that you already exercise on a regular basis. If you don't, then shame on you! If you need only one good reason to exercise - it reduces stress. Let me repeat that. It reduces stress.

Exercise helps you maintain a healthy weight; helps you sleep better; makes you happier and healthier; increases your life expectancy; and prevents debilitating and deadly diseases like cancer, stroke, heart disease and diabetes. Just get moving and do it. No excuses. Keep in mind that it is strongly recommended that you consult with your doctor before starting any exercise routine.

If you're struggling to exercise on a regular basis it might be because you haven't found something you enjoy. Let's be realistic here. If you join a gym, but you hate going, you're not going to go. However, if you find something you enjoy doing you'll look forward to it instead of dreading it. There are many, many things to choose from.

Here's a short list of options:

Walking
Running
Hiking
Cross-country skiing
Tennis
Yoga
Pilates
Dance classes

Strength training
Kickboxing
Zumba
Spinning
Surfing
Paddle boarding
Swimming

There is an amazing plethora of free videos on YouTube to choose from. If you like to work out in the comfort of your own home just do that. It doesn't matter what you do, as long as you get your heart pumping and you feel good. If you need motivation find a workout buddy.
Someone you look forward to talking to.

Now let's get you zipping up and looking hot in that dress. Here's what you have to do: burn more calories than you normally do. Regardless of what you are currently doing for exercise, you need to find ways to get at least an extra 10 minutes of exercise in every day. It's just 10 minutes. Again, this is only for one week. But you can use these ways to squeeze in exercise anytime. Or even just on really busy days when you don't have time to get in a full workout. The next chapter will show you ways to squeeze in exercise even on busy days.

Chapter 7
How to Squeeze in Exercise
On Busy Days

Sometimes our days are so jam packed that we can't even imagine getting a workout in. But I find that even a short run rather than no run at all can make all the difference in my day. That 10 minutes alone of fresh air and exercise can alter my day by relieving stress and reducing the guilt factor of not working out.

There is no question that ideally taking an hour to run, work your core and arms (push-ups or whatever) or grab a yoga class, or go to the gym (whatever you do for exercise) is the best way to exercise. But let's face it - it isn't always possible. Plus, are you really going to sweat so much in 10 minutes that you'll need a shower? Or even need to change your clothes?

Here are 10 ways to squeeze in exercise even on the busiest days:

1. Get up earlier in the morning. Nothing gets your metabolism going faster than getting your blood flowing first thing in the morning. Even if it's just a quick 10-minute abdominal video or some squats and pushups followed by stretching. You'll not only feel great physically, but you'll be proud of yourself for doing it.

2. Exercise while watching TV at night or in the evening. You can do arm exercises with light weights or a resistance band. Or try taking your lazy tush off the couch and sit on a balance ball

while watching your favorite show. Mix it up and get creative. You'll burn extra calories and not feel guilty if you need a nighttime snack.

3. Take the stairs. Take the stairs instead of the elevator whenever possible. This is a great way to burn more calories. Plus, climbing stairs is perfect for toning the thighs, calves and glutes (that's your gluteus maximus aka buttocks).

4. Dance. Dancing is another way to burn extra calories. And it's fun. Throw on some music and dance while you do the dishes. My kids and I will often have a cleanup dance party. Or just throw on some music and dance in the family room for a while.

5. Walk whenever you can. Park your car far away from the entrance in the parking lot while running errands. But don't do this at night or if the parking lot is deserted. Safety always takes precedence over exercise.

6. Spread out your workout into intervals throughout the day. Try something like this: 10 minutes of core in the morning; walking during your lunch break or right after work; three quick sets of pushups while dinner is in the oven; jump rope while watching television.

7. This is a little trick I learned from a supermodel. Years ago, I was watching some talk show and the host asked an older but famous supermodel, how she keeps in shape. I honestly can't remember which model it was but that's irrelevant. Her

response was that she does exercises while doing other things. She does side skaters while blowing her hair dry. Work out and get stuff done at the same time? Genius! Multi-tasking. I have been doing this ever since. When I brush my teeth or scrub my face, I do knee lifts to work my core. If I'm watching an educational video for research, I grab the weights and work my arms. When I fill my water glass from the cold filtered refrigerator, I do side or back leg lifts and/or squats. If you're doing something where you can't be moving around just crouch yourself into a yoga chair pose. Driving? Butt crunches, Kegels and thigh squeezes. You might look silly while you're doing it. But when someone looks at you and says, "Wow. Do you work out every day?" You can
say, "Why yes. Yes, I do."

8. Exercise while you're sitting. This goes along with the multitasking idea. If you spend a lot of time sitting whether it be for work, taking an online class or get stuck sitting while traveling, there are still ways to squeeze in exercise. Try sitting on a balance ball. If you sit up straight and tighten your tummy you can engage your core building strength in your abdominals, obliques and back. Do butt crunches and inner thigh squeezes. They're easy to do and can get your thighs and glutes toned fast. And it burns calories!

9. HIIT. High Intensity Interval Training is a cardiovascular exercise that alternates intense spurts of exercise with less intense recovery periods. You can incorporate this into many

different exercises from running, jumping rope or weight training.

10. Here's a quick HIIT workout I do when I only have 20 minutes, but I want something intense. Walk for 2 minutes, run at a slow to moderate pace for 2 minutes, run fast for 2 minutes.
Repeat 3 times.

Chapter 8
Ten Tricks to Help You Lose Weight

There are many little things you can do, on a daily basis and throughout the day to help you lose weight fast. They are simple and probably nothing you haven't already heard before. But if you were doing them, then you probably wouldn't be reading my book. So even if this is just a reminder for you, then this is the week to focus on those little things that can really add up.

1. Drink an entire glass of water before each meal. This will fill you up and prevent you from eating as much.

2. Drink a lot of water throughout the day. All day. Always have a glass of water nearby. Keep a glass by your bed. Keep a water cup in the bathroom. Always bring water in the car. And if you cook a lot and spend a lot of time in the kitchen like I do, always have a glass of water handy on the kitchen counter. I even go so far as to grab a cup or bottle of water at the grocery store from the cafe, while I'm shopping. Stay hydrated.

3. If you feel hungry try drinking a glass of water first. Sometimes your body tricks you into thinking you're hungry when you're really, just thirsty. If you're still hungry after you drink the water, have a snack.

4. Eat spicy food. It fills you up and keeps you feeling full longer. I personally love spicy food and like to put crushed red pepper and/or hot sauce on almost everything. Be careful with the hot sauce though

because they usually contain a lot of salt. If you don't like spicy food or your taste buds (or tummy) can't handle it - then just skip this. No biggie.

5. In place of a midafternoon snack, enjoy a warm cup of tea or decaf coffee. It will fill you up even it's just temporary and will hold you over to the next snack.

6. Snack, snack, snack. Snacking is healthy. It keeps your metabolism active throughout the day and prevents you from eating larger meals.

7. Don't snack after 9pm. When you eat closer to your bedtime it leaves less time to burn off the calories. Plus, a short fasting period can be healthy and promote weight loss. However, this is NOT a rule but a guideline. If you are really hungry, and need a bedtime snack, it's okay. Especially if you had a long or intense workout, that day. You might need the extra calories to sustain you through the night. But keep it small and choose your snack wisely. Because you're going low carb this week try a small handful of nuts or a little plain Greek yogurt.

8. Eat smaller portions and smaller meals. You've heard this before. You don't need to pile a ton of food onto your plate. Eat a lighter meal to start. Then wait a little bit to see if you're still hungry. Sometimes it takes a while for your brain to register that you're full. If you decide you need more to eat, have more vegetables.

9. As a rule, and whenever possible, try sitting instead of lying down, standing instead of sitting, walking

instead of standing. It might not seem like much, but every little bit adds up and every calorie you burn counts.

10. Bring healthy snacks with you. I try to always keep nuts or healthy snacks in the car. You'll avoid the drive thru where you'll be tempted to get sugary drinks or unhealthy food like muffins or donuts. Cut up veggies ahead of time and put them in individual sized containers so you can grab them and go (to save time cut up extra when you're making them for breakfast, lunch or dinner). FYI - muffins are cake in cute little individual portions.

Chapter 9
Healthy Morning Habits

The morning is an extremely important part of your day. It can set the tone for the whole day and either set you up for success or failure. It can also be a crazy part of the day. Especially if you have children, you're getting ready for work, preparing to travel or just have a busy day ahead. Creating healthy morning habits will help you succeed whether you're trying to lose weight, maintain a healthy weight or other goals in life.

Morning is often my favorite part of the day. Especially when I get up early, before everyone else in the house, and everything is quiet. I've put together some healthy morning habits that work for me or that I've tried over the years. I hope you get at least one new idea out of this chapter and it works for you too.

Here are 8 healthy morning habits you can try:

1. Drink water. The first thing you should do in the morning is drink a glass of water. Your body becomes dehydrated while sleeping. It will energize you and stave off hunger. Sometimes when you feel hungry you are actually thirsty. You can tell if you're dehydrated by the color of your urine. It should be mostly clear with a tinge of yellow. If it is dark yellow, you should drink a glass of water. Dry lips, dry skin, muscle cramps and headaches are also signs of dehydration.

2. Be thankful. I like to start my day thinking about what I'm thankful for. It might sound silly, but it creates a positive mindset that will help you achieve your goals.

3. Enjoy something warm. There's nothing better than starting the day with a warm cup of tea or coffee. Especially on a chilly morning. If you don't "do caffeine" have a cup of herbal tea or warm water with lemon.

4. Take vitamins. Taking a daily multivitamin supplement ensures that you are getting the recommended daily value of vitamins your body needs to be healthy. If you're not sure whether you should take vitamin supplements, consult your doctor.

5. Read. I like to start my day reading the latest health and fitness news. It doesn't feel like work to me because I enjoy it. Read something you enjoy whether it's the newspaper, a magazine or inspirational book.

6. Meditate. Meditation reduces stress, improves concentration and encourages a healthy lifestyle.

7. Exercise. If you exercise first thing in the morning, there will be less chance of something coming up to prevent you from exercising. Morning exercise also energizes you, reduces stress and makes you feel good. Physically and mentally.

8. Eat a healthy breakfast. Breakfast is the most important meal of the day. It gives you energy and revs up your metabolism to start burning calories. Starting the day with a healthy breakfast will also set the tone for a day of healthy eating.

Chapter 10
Eight Old-School Weight Loss Tips

This won't be the first time you've heard these tried and true methods to help you lose weight. And it won't be the last. That's because they work. Despite every new trend that comes and goes, you can never lose by going back to the basics.

Here's a short list of simple and effective ways to lose weight:

1. Exercise. Find a workout buddy or exercise with a group. Most excuses I hear for not exercising boil down to one thing - motivation. It doesn't matter what you say, if you were motivated to exercise you would do it. Having a friend, you enjoy spending time with or meeting with a group can help motivate you. Or guilt you when you don't show up. If it's motivation you need, find a group class or a friend to workout with. Most importantly, make it fun so you look forward to it rather than dreading it.

2. Avoid processed foods. Processed foods often contain unnecessary sodium, fat and sugar. If it's convenience you're looking for, read the labels. Avoid anything that is high in sodium or contains high fructose corn syrup.

3. Cook at home. Cooking at home ensures that you know what you're eating. Prepare fresh all naturals foods. You can control what you put into your food by cooking with olive oil and omitting (or reducing) the amount of salt and sugar that goes into a recipe. I almost always reduce the amount of salt,

fat (butter or oil) and sugar that goes into a recipe and almost never notice a difference.

4. Eat low fat dairy products. Obviously, this won't work for you if you are vegan. But if you do eat dairy, it can fill you up and give you much needed protein. Plain Greek yogurt and cottage cheese make great snack foods. Another healthy snack is a glass of skim milk with a banana. Try a teaspoon of almond butter on your banana if you need a little more substance.

5. Limit your sugar intake. Reducing sugar has been linked to weight loss for a long time. It is high in calories and provides no nutritional value. Most foods that contain sugar are also high in fat like donuts, cake and cookies. Think moderation when it comes to these sweet treats.

6. Track what you eat. If you eat mindlessly, writing down what you eat can be beneficial. You might be surprised at what you find. It can also help you determine what foods sustain you and keep you full longer. This encourage healthier snacking and reducing overall food intake.

7. Avoid artificial sweeteners. They are linked to weight gain and cancer. Diet sodas and other foods marked as "diet foods" can be misleading. Read labels and be careful with what you put into your body. All-natural foods are always best.

8. Avoid or limit alcohol. Alcohol is filled with empty calories and is often combined with high calorie sugary mixers. It also metabolizes faster than food which hinders weight loss. The effects of alcohol lower your inhibitions making you more likely to

indulge in foods you might otherwise stay away from. If you do have alcohol, choose a glass a wine, a light beer or a low-calorie mixer such as club soda.

Chapter 11
Crunch Time

If your goal was indeed to lose weight, so you can look great in a hot little dress, then that day will eventually come. Or if you'll be soaking up the rays by the pool. Whatever your motivation, it doesn't just stop here. At this point you should be (and I certainly hope you are) feeling pretty good about yourself. If you need a little added incentive, remind yourself that tonight you're going to have a good time and maybe even enjoy a few cocktails. Or maybe have a little dessert.

Today however is not the day to blow it. You don't want to feel bloated. The night before the day of the event (or before you're about to hop on a plane) I would try not to eat anything past 7 pm or at least a couple of hours before you go to bed. If you're feeling hungry try a nice cup of warm herbal tea with lemon.

On the morning of the event squeeze half of a lemon (or lime) into 8 ounces of water and drink the entire glass. Then continue to drink lemon water throughout the day. This will prevent and/or reduce bloating.

Stick with what has been working for you over the past week. Continue to eat lean protein and lots of vegetables. Eat small meals and snack throughout the day.

The worst thing you can do at this point is to go to the event or on vacation and now completely blow everything you've just done. Hopefully, you'll feel so good, you won't have the desire to indulge in the basket of rolls circling around the table. Then finishing your own dessert before digging into the one left untouched, by someone out on the dance floor.

I'm not saying not to reward yourself. But why would you go through all this trouble only to put it all back on again in a day or two?

Make it a priority today, to get in a good workout. Whatever you decide to do make sure it involves some cardio, abdominal exercises and arms. In fact, I usually do a set of push-ups right before I go out. *Especially* if I'm wearing a sexy strappy dress. Yes, I will literally get down on my family room floor in my cocktail dress and do sets of push-ups. It really tones up your arms for a spectacular evening of complements at the event. This is a secret I've been keeping for years. Now I'm sharing it with you.

Chapter 12
Keeping the Weight Off

It is my sincere hope that you feel great and want to keep the weight off. You should feel good every day. But life is short and one of the many pleasures in life is indulging in delicious food. It's important to ease back into a well-balanced diet filled with nutritious fruit, vegetables, lean protein, nuts, legumes and whole grains.

Keep eating the foods you've been enjoying this past week and stick with the habits that have worked for you. Hopefully, by now you don't even miss some of the sweet sugary foods. If you start to put on weight just go back to this for a day or two, to get back on track.

Here are some ways to help you keep weight off and maintain a healthy weight:

1. Weigh yourself every day. This is controversial and yes, it's also important to notice how you feel in your clothes. But weighing yourself every day keeps you in check. Even if it is water weight. You can think about what you ate the day before that may have been processed or high in sodium, that you should not eat again. Or what great workout you did. That despite the dessert you ate last night is showing a loss on the scale. But most importantly, if you don't weigh yourself for a while you might jump on the scale and have gained 5 pounds. It's way harder to take the weight off than it is to put in on.

2. Continue to exercise on a regular basis. Find something that you enjoy doing and look forward

to. If you hate doing it, you won't keep it up. If you get bored just find something else that you like doing. It's healthy to mix in a variety of exercise like walking, running, bike riding, weight lifting, yoga, or Pilates. There are so many choices that there's no excuse.

3. Eat a healthy well-balanced diet.

4. Reward yourself. It's okay to treat yourself but make good choices. Have a small bowl of ice cream or whatever, rather than eating out of the carton and devouring the entire thing. It's also better to have a treat early in the day so you have all day to burn off the calories. It will satisfy your craving and prevent you from binging later in the day.

5. Eat breakfast. If the morning is rushed or you typically aren't hungry first thing in the morning, that's okay. Just eat a light breakfast mid-morning. But don't skip it altogether. I often don't eat breakfast until I've been up for a couple of hours.

6. Work out first thing in the morning. This isn't always the easiest thing in the world to do but try when you can. There's less chance of something coming up during the day that will prevent you from working out at all.

7. Exercise every day (or most days) for at least 10 minutes. It may not be ideal but every bit of exercise counts. Plus, it's fun to do different short spurts of exercise.

8. Don't beat yourself up if you have a bad day of
    eating or don't exercise. It will only discourage you.
    Just do better the next day.

Like anything in life, you must truly want something in life
to achieve it. My kudos to you for sticking through this,
looking fabulous in that little black dress and committing
yourself to living a longer and healthier life.

Disclaimer

This book does not provide medical advice. **You should consult your physician before beginning any exercise, weight loss or health care program.** This book **should not** be used as a replacement for a visit to a competent healthcare professional. You should consult a physician before adapting any of the suggestions in this book or before drawing inferences from it.

Results May Vary: Causes for being overweight or obese vary from person to person. Whether genetic or environmental, it should be noted that food intake, rates of metabolism and levels of exercise and physical exertion vary from person to person. This means weight loss results will also vary from person to person. No individual result should be seen as typical.

The statements in this book are of opinion and not medically proven. The information is not intended in any way as a substitute for professional medical advice. Always seek the advice of your physician or other qualified healthcare provider with any questions you may have regarding weight loss.

About the Author

Irene Gabelnick is a health and fitness blogger. She has been an avid runner most of her life. She enjoys hiking, bouldering, mountain biking, doing yoga, Pilates, strength training, skydiving and she even surfed the crazy waves in Hawaii!

Discover how to feel confident in everything you wear. *Or nothing at all...* Learn more at irenegabelnick.com.